The Alchemy of Yoga:
Living Yoga off the Mat

Wendy Reese Hartmann

ISBN-13: 978-0692784433 (Whole Being Inc)

Photographs by: Red Bird Photography, http://www.redbirdphotography.org/

DEDICATION

In memory of
Michael and Wayne.

In honor of
yoga students everywhere.

TABLE OF CONTENTS

FOREWARD

I never meant to teach yoga.
Yoga found me.
And along the journey
of the past 15 years,
I've learned a few things
that come from a soulful longing
of something more than the asanas.

This is my yogic wisdom and these are my stories.
Or at least how I have defined them.
It's also the wisdom and stories of my Guides…
at least as best as I can tell.

Memory is a tricky thing —
we forget what we want to remember
remember what we want to forget
and change the facts to remember ourselves as a better version
of reality.

At any rate, there's a lot to remember;
seems this life isn't my first rodeo.
Been here before.
But I'm not one to admit to believing in reincarnation.
Whatever I am, contradiction is a great starting description.

Over the years, I have come to know yoga
as so much more than a physical exercise
(although it is excellent for that)
but as wisdom for living off the mat:
balance, strength, flexibility, and surrender.
It's given me a safe place to remember
my deepest knowing and truest Self.

My biggest hope is that someone will pick this up
give it a read
and feel the jolt of remembrance:
the reason why they're here
their power
and the knowledge of choice.
Because if they can, they can short cut their way to the front of the "enlightenment" line
and play on a scale few have been willing to play on here on Earth.
If enough do,
things change.
And oh, how we need a change.

Part 1

The Alchemy of Yoga

Give me an hour, I'll give you peace. Guess that makes me a bit of a bliss-pusher. Cheaper, healthier, and more legal than drugs. I'm a yoga teacher. Over the past fifteen years I have watched many students come into class stressed out and leave blissed out.

If you've done yoga more than a few times, you know the cycle I'm talking about. There is no one-size-fits-all reason for all that bliss happening in yoga though. Maybe you were on your game physically, you released some stress, you experienced feeling again, or something else, a deeper connection to your whole being.

The roots of the bliss probably reside in the definition of yoga itself. Yoga means union. But have you ever wondered union with what?

Yourself?

Your body?

Your breath?

Source/God/Divine/Universe?

Other people?

Something else?

Nothingness?

Consciousness?

Your shadows and light?

The present?

Your Truth?

I've never heard the question effectively answered. I think the answer lies in a reframe of the question. What do *you* want to unite with? For me as a teacher *and* student, it has become a combination of all of those and then some.

At the start of a yoga practice, I just want to unite with the present moment—

let go of all the good and the bad that may (or may not) have happened since the last time I stepped on the mat (which is often too long between practices). To do that, I have to unite with my breath and intention.

Be here now.

Inhaling, "I am."

Exhaling, "here now."

Because now is all we have, but few of us live like that. Do you?

When we move through the practice, we try to unite with our body.

What's our body telling us in the present moment of now?

Where are we strong?

Where are we weak?

Where are we compensating?

Where are our boundaries?

Where do we need more attention, more breath, more patience?

More acceptance?

I have seen how quickly an illness, injury, or life event can derail a person and affect the body. What you could do yesterday, you might not be able to do today and who knows when you'll do it again… or it. Then again, perhaps you'll do it better. You just never know until you show up on the mat.

That's where union with acceptance is critical. Without it, we become self-judgmental, critical, and ego-driven. That can (and often does) lead to more injuries. For me, just knowing where my body is tight or tired allows me to set healthy boundaries. I create safety for myself. Nobody knows our bodies better than ourselves. Even if a teacher sees where we could improve our asana, it doesn't necessarily mean we should do that adjustment.

And yet, we (or many of us) take our teachers instructions as the end all. If the instructor is experienced, educated, intuitive, and empathic, they probably can read your body pretty well, but they can't *know* 100% how you're feeling.

I didn't listen to my inner wisdom until I was faced with a serious injury that took a long time to heal. I had no choice to listen to my body if I wanted to avoid re-injury. If a correction wasn't appropriate for me, I told the teacher, "Thank you, that just won't work for me right now." Most teachers respect that and your body will, too!

More often than not, my teachers' have made for assists me that provide more freedom to deepen the asana. Personally, I appreciate those assists. When I am practicing, I am constantly focusing on my alignment. The brain is a workhorse eager to do the asana practice. The alignment cues give my mind something to work on:

root down through the four corners of the feet

soften the knees

shift the inner thighs back

slightly draw in and up two inches below the belly button

open and relax the low back

draw back the ribs, broadening the middle back

roll the collarbones back slightly

bring the chin parallel to the floor

draw the ears over the shoulders

grow taller.

About the time I get to the top, I realize I've lost the foundation and have to start again. I am continually beginning again. Feels a lot like life off the mat, too. Always, we begin again.

After a while, the mind and body unite. My head and body co-habitats in the same zip code for an ever-so-short period of time. Have you ever felt like your mind is about a block away from your body, completely disconnected, even if still attached? When we focus on the alignment continuously, all that stuff our brain had been focused on gets pushed aside in order to stay present and aligned. It's awesome.

There is a fine line, though. At some point I have to stop doing and start being in the asana. Allow my mind to become calm and steady through the breath. Allow my body to be still. Trust me when I say that is harder than all the adjustments, yet it is the most necessary. That's why we practice. So that off the mat we we can find a steadiness in life even when the world around us feels chaotic.

By the end of a practice, I unite with sweet surrender. Nothing to do or fix, just BE. I am uniting for a few sweet moments with All That Is, peace, and possibility.

During *savasana* (corpse pose), I have received sparks of inspiration, solutions to problems, profound peace, and plenty of visits from the dead— some I have known and some who saw me as a channel. It's interesting, to say the least.

If I am teaching, I am uniting with the students. What are their bodies and energy telling me? What are their souls telling me? What are my guides telling me? Therefore, I am also uniting with the supernatural, my inner wisdom, and the Mystery of it all.

Guiding *savasana*, when I walk around with aromatherapy and massage students' foreheads, scalps, and earlobes, I unite with unconditional love. I don't care who they are, what they've done or left undone, where they're going or how they'll get there. I just know in that moment, like all moments, they deserve unconditional love and I am willing to give it.

I strive to unite my bliss and peace that I find on the mat into my world *off* the mat. The beginning and ending of my day are designed to help me unite with my Highest-Self. I try my best to unite to my deepest wisdom, compassion, and love daily. Most days, at best, I graze it. Still, I have to keep showing up, keep being willing to BE me, united, congruent, whole.

There is a school of yoga, Shaviate Tantra, that believes that we are all a piece of the Divine Feminine and Masculine who came to Earth in human form to contract into limitations; a contrast of their Truth. They do this as Divine Play. Once in the contraction, they must expand back into their unlimited wholeness.

Now, if that's true, we are all a piece of the same cloth, just living out our own version of the contractions and expansions through our experience of shadows and light within ourselves and others.

That's the whole interconnected Oneness hippy-dippy-New-Age-hold-hands-singing-Kumbaya part of yoga. Even if we all hold a piece of this Divinity within, Consciousness wants to evolve. It does that through each of us and our own unique experiences. In other words, in this very moment, everything is as it should be. It's perfect. Yes, even *that.* Most of us don't see everything as perfect.

Here's the deal, though. What we judge about others is a reflection of some fear or self-judgment of ourselves. Alas, the union with others is a stepping stone to uniting with ourselves. We *need* each other to complete that journey. Union with other to have union with our Self. Deep.

That's the kind of stuff that sounds all wonderful until you're facing a murderer, dictator, pedophile, greedy CEO willing to overlook the environment or humanity to make more money. You might find yourself exclaiming, "I'm not them. No way! I could never!"

Why not? How do you know? Having not been in the same shoes, *how do you know*? We simply do not know what their deeper purpose is. For all we know it could be their desired growth experience or the growth of someone else, including humanity. Just because things are perfect as is doesn't mean there isn't a potential for a *different* perfection. Consciousness evolving. We have to be willing to see the shadows and light are in us to know the shadows and light in them aren't as black and white as we originally thought.

That's where the work of the asanas really start coming off the mat.

Union of:

acceptance

presence

what's alive in me, in others

mind and body

the supernatural

inner wisdom

the Mystery of it all

surrender

BEing

That's just the beginning.

Why did you first go to a yoga class? Perhaps it was it to:

recover from illness or injury

be more flexible

cross train

lose weight

decrease stress

prevent injury

find peace

heal.

Just as there are many reasons to step on the mat, there are an equally large variety of styles (and teachers) to choose from. I was taught Hatha yoga with an Anusara influence. It suits me. As an Exercise Science major in college, I was trained to work with body mechanics. I am a body geek. My background provides me a unique way to look at someone's body. I can help them find more space to make asanas freer, though not necessarily easier. This freedom allows them to explore the asana at a deeper level than they would have been able to while fighting to sculpt their body into something that wasn't working.

The reasons people stay with yoga are even more unique than the reason they came. Yoga is alchemy. If you are willing to stick with it, yoga changes you. Perhaps it's that you start to feel again or those deeply buried parts are able to finally be healed. Personally, I think we find acceptance and that allows the parts of us we've hidden away for safe keeping to unite and we align more closely with our true self. I know how woo-woo that sounds, but I have enough proof to know the truth of that.

For just a little while, whatever notion you have of yoga — beautiful, tightly clad, green-juice drinking, vegan women or the bearded man-bun wearing, six-pack donning male yogis chanting and touting a life of rainbow and unicorns — forget that bullshit for a minute. I've seen those people, but not typically in *my* classes.

I see men and women who wonder why they're still alive, if they can make it through the day, or how they'll make it through the month. They've seen amazing and crazy things throughout their lives. They also have loved deeply, been hurt badly, and somehow can't quite give up. I've seen corporate people, parents, high school and college students, retirees, veterans, singles, couples, divorcees, and widows. All ages, races, religions (including atheist), sexual preferences, and genders. I've even had students who transitioned genders.

We've laughed, explored, cried, brainstormed, regrouped, reflected, and cheered each other on over the years. I've even married some of my students. Okay, they got married, I just officiated. There have been plenty of babies (aka future students) arrive and I always feel that they should be the teachers because they know how to just be; open, trusting, simple, pure, and free from all the conditioning adults bring to the mat. And, as with life, some students have died (not doing yoga), which was sad and hard and truly sucked, but they've never left my heart.

As *you* know, yoga is not just for the young, beautiful, healthy people of this world. That's just selling it short. Yoga teaches us how to be flexible. It makes us stronger. It improves our balance. And it encourages us to surrender our ego and pride. All traits that are highly beneficial off the mat, too. Let's start with flexibility.

Flexibility

The conversation often goes like this:

"So what do you do?"

"I teach yoga."

"Oh. I don't do yoga because I'm not flexible."

You don't do yoga because you are flexible. You do yoga to *become* flexible.

Inflexibility transcends the muscles and reflects the rigidity of the mind. Seriously. Rigidity comes from a place of fearing judgment, abandonment, or being unloved. Have you ever experienced a time when you showed up authentically and experienced being judged, shunned, or treated harshly? That hurts. It is natural to avoid hurt. When you avoid hurt, play it safe, you become rigid.

The mind is like a computer; it creates a file for every experience. Humans like the good feeling stuff and naturally want more of it. The mind works hard to try to protect the "user" (aka human) from experiencing hurt. The brain has a built-in search engine that references past experiences to determine what to avoid in the present. This leads to taking fewer risks. It also eliminates the infinite possibilities in the present moment. Ultimately, it is fear based living— inflexible and limited.

People often define themselves as inflexible when their hamstrings, low back, or shoulders are tight. As a teacher, I see (with the exception of genetics or traumatic injuries):

tight hamstrings most often in people who have struggled with feeling safe and secure;

tight shoulders in people who have struggled with authenticity — shapeshifting in order to be accepted and loved or withholding their truth in order to feel safe;

tight lower backs associated with relationship (both past and present) and money issues.

When a fear is triggered and the need arises to control the outcome of a situation, the low back will tense. It's hard to trust — the Universe, other people, even ourselves — when we're fearful. When the mind constantly tries to protect us from painful experiences, we struggle to trust the intuitive urge to explore, go deeper, surrender into authenticity. Easier to stay on the edges, playing it safe.

I have spent entire classes working on various forward folds to open the hamstrings and low back. The intention was to expand flexibility, build self-trust, and explore safety and security. With both feet firmly rooted onto the mat in *uttinasana*, standing forward fold, you can discover a place of support and safety.

Start the *uttinasana* by bending the knees and practicing compassion by supporting the hamstrings, not overly stretching them. Slowly and mindfully, straighten the legs. Each time you bend your knees and gently straighten them, you practice self-trust and honor the body by asking your body, "Where do you want to open in this moment and do you feel supported enough to do that?"

I ask the class to honor what they feel, adding supports as needed, removing them as they feel comfortable. The more flexible their legs became, the more length their spine achieved, making the pose both flexible *and* strong. They found more space and less resistance in their own body.

I started to notice something interesting in both myself and the students. As we continue to practice self-trust and self-compassion on the mat, our bodies becoming more flexible, it correlates off the mat. We become more gentle and patient with ourselves and others, willing to trust our intuition, and to take more risks in being vulnerable.

An exploration on the mat of "what else is there?" led me to a journey of infinite possibilities off the mat. I no longer approached life rigidly; black or white, good or bad, dark or light, right or wrong. Within each experience, I saw the complexity of people, places, and things.

I discovered that I could hold a space for love even with people I neither liked, nor agreed with in our world views. With the people I was closer to who traditionally triggered me, I started setting healthy boundaries. They had the right to their own beliefs and rigidity, but I didn't have to play on that playground with them anymore. I started playing different games, more loving and joyful. As my energy elevated, I noticed they either tried to pull me down or avoided me all together. When they couldn't pull me down, they walked away. Misery loves company and I was no longer good company.

What was interesting was I started attracting new people into my life who vibrated at a similar or higher energy, fueling my momentum. As I continued to explore and soften my outer (formerly hardened) edges, I opened into possibilities. Curiosity and playfulness overtook the space where fear had driven my thoughts and beliefs.

Every shoulder stretch, forward fold, and backbend opened my heart and mind a little more. The more I listened to my body's needs, the more self-trust I established. That translated off the mat, too. I began to notice I wasn't taking things so personally, either. I started dropping the stories I made up about my experience and started searching for factual data.

Begin to challenge yourself by asking "I wonder if that's really true?" every time you find a difficult asana that scares you or you think you can't do. Take the question off the mat for anything you think impossible or unlikely. Most of the time, it will only partially true, if at all. Your world on and off the mat will expand vastly with each challenge.

As I became more "bendy," I weathered the storms that came and went in my life with greater ease. I would ask with curiosity, "I wonder what the lesson is here? Why would I choose *this* experience, consciously or subconsciously?" Just like when I would lean into my inflexible places on the mat, I would simply deepen my breath and listen, exploring what was there in that moment, in that space.

Sometimes I could find more space to explore and sometimes I would hit my resistance and back off.

In those later moments, I always knew that if I was willing to return at some point things would likely be different. They usually were. Just because you hit the wall in one moment, doesn't mean you'll always hit the wall. It's just a moment and that moment changes quickly. We simply need to return to the breath and be willing to listen. The flexibility will be there when it's time. The question is, will you?

Flexibility starts by being willing to show up and explore. It takes strength to show up, again and again. If you're willing to show up, we can start exploring how to develop the strength needed to keep showing up.

Toolbox

Now it's your turn to integrate it. Read through and then give it a try. You don't have to be perfect, just try it. You can see photos and receive additional tools on the resource page of my website at www.wholebeinginc.com/toolbox. This page is for the people who have purchased the book only. Your own secret into my yoga goodness, so please hold it close to your heart and refrain from sharing. (Remember, karma knows.)

Asana: postures mentioned in this chapter

Uttinasana

Stand with feet hip distance apart. Lift your toes. Notice how that connects the four corners of your feet to the floor while lifting the arches of the feet. Maintain that lift as you spread the toes before lightly returning to the floor. Soften the knees. Inhale and reach the arms out to the sides and up to the ceiling. Bring the palms to touch. As you lower the hands to the heart, bow forward, lengthening the spine as you reach the hands down to a block or the ground. Keep the weight on the balls of the feet. The goal is to maintain as straight a spine as possible. Keep the softness in the knees or bend deeper if your hamstrings are tight and the spine curves.

With each inhalation, bring the awareness to your low back. Imagine you can send your breath there to create expansion as you lengthen the spine ever so slightly. As you exhale, move the inner thighs back and up slightly, drawing the belly in and upwards (toward the ribs). Hold for five slow breaths before bringing palms to the tops of thighs, lengthening the spine, pressing feet down to return to a standing position.

Janu Sirsasana

Sitting on the floor, one leg extended in front of you, the other bent with the foot on the inner thigh of the extended leg. (You can place a blanket or block under the bent knee to support it) Place your hands on the floor behind your hips, stretch upward. Use a strap around the ball of the foot or place hands on shin or around bottom of foot. Reach heart towards the foot of the extended leg. Inhale and back out of the pose by 10% to lengthen spine more, exhale, drawing the belly slightly in and up to go slightly deeper into the pose. Try to open the space in the chest by drawing the shoulders back and slightly together. Hold for five slow breaths before returning to the starting position and switching sides.

Swadhyaya: self-exploration

Rooting down

In both of these asanas, the connection to the earth before exploring your boundaries in flexibility is very important. In life, being "grounded" or "centered" provides a safe place to start exploring the parts of you ready to shift. What makes you feel "rooted"? How can you connect more deeply in your rootedness?

Drawing inward

To become more flexible, you have to be willing to listen to yourself. What do you need? What feedback is your body offering? Intuition will sometimes use words, but if you haven't been listening, it will more likely use a contracted or expansive sensation to give you a "no" or "yes" respectively. When you move beyond your physical flexibility, your body will always let you know. If you ignore it and keep pushing, you'll probably experience an injury. The same holds true off the mat. Do you listen to yourself?

Find the edges and back off

Do you trust what you hear or do you try to muscle your way through? How often do you deny yourself basic needs just to get a little more done? What would happen if you backed off even 10%? How would that feel and what would change?

Follow the breath

The breath brings us back to the present moment. It gives us a pause to check-in and see what is possible in that moment. Doing this gives us an opportunity to experience the moment in its uniqueness rather than how we expect or desire it to be. Do you notice your breath? Is it short and shallow or deep and steady?

Safety, acceptance, love

Once our basic needs are met (food, water, shelter), we start trying to meet our emotional basic needs. What makes you feel safe, accepted, and loved? Are you able to accept yourself, take care of your needs, and love yourself? Or do you constantly seek others to meet those needs?

Pranayam: breath work

Try extending your breath by exhaling twice as long as the inhale. If you inhale for two seconds, exhale for four.

Mudra: gestures of the hand that shift physical and mental states

Prithivi Mudra

With the palms facing up, touch the tip of the thumb to the ring finger with light pressure. This mudra helps to increase strength and groundedness, restores equilibrium and trust.

Mantra: an affirmation to anchor desired shift

I am willing to listen and trust my deepest wisdom.

Strength

The class transitioned between sun salutation to *Virabadrasana* I, or Warrior I. My intention was to do three rounds of *Virabadrasana* I on each side, transitioning to each side through a sun salutation. The first round would be for alignment. The second would be to find more space and practice surrendering resistance and ego. The final round would be to find the fullest expression of the asana.

Looking at the students standing in warrior, facing forward with their arms raised, something dawned on me. This asana represents courage. Their legs were in the yogic version of a boxers stance. All seven major chakras faced forward, fully exposed. In that moment, I saw how vulnerable this asana is considering its name. Though I am continually encouraging students to listen to and follow their hearts deepest desires, I realized it takes courage to show up fully, authentically, with integrity, love, compassion, to do the right thing when it's not the popular thing.

I heard the words coming through me, out of my mouth but not mine: "You have to have courage to raise your arms and send out the love and light from your heart. Bring the hands together in Kali mudra. Kali is the Hindu goddess who cuts through anything that is no longer serving. What are you ready to cut through in your life in order to be courageously you? Three breaths here." I walked around the room, my energy suddenly bigger, stronger like I was channeling the Goddess Kali herself.

I took them through a sun salutation to transition to the other side. "Hands to Kali mudra, lift the heart up this time. You are strong, courageous and wise. You are powerful and mighty. Feel that now. Engage that strength to sever what no longer serves us. Remember your own strength to stand grounded in your Truth, to be authentic, to do what is right even when the risk is high."

Mental fortitude and strength are every bit as important as physical fortitude and strength in our daily living. For these are the qualities that are continually tested by our lives - through work, relationships, health, esteem, decisions, goals, dreams and desires.

It doesn't matter what you do. There's nothing left *to do* really. Action is the Divine Masculine at play. Being is Divine Feminine at play. Strength comes from a balance of both, not just the doing.

What matters is *why* you show up, play, and be. Think about a time you went to yoga class and tried to push yourself when your body just wasn't in a place to be pushed. The class was probably much harder than it needed to be. Now think of a time when you were just happy to be there, didn't care how well you did, or were surprised by how well you did. That's the difference between doing and being.

You have to be willing to move through the questions and actually become the questions; feel how they feel on your skin, taste on your tongue, smell in your nose, sound in your ears, and look through your eyes. Feel the questions. Sense the questions. Don't just think about the answers.

In thinking, you can find yourself wishing away and regretting or resenting everything. You can even kill yourself if you get desperate enough to end the suffering. But you cannot abolish what *is*. You are. I am. We are. You can end the finite body, but you cannot end the infinite. You can destroy your ability to speak your Truth, but not your potential. You did not create yourself and try as you might, you cannot destroy the Divine Intelligence within you. Therefore, we must courageously explore who that is and why It is here now.

Reflect on all the ways you have held your purest potential back by playing small and doing what you needed to do to survive. The problem is in surviving; you played small long enough that the fears became beliefs and the beliefs dictated your life. You become lost because of a bad internal GPS. Feeling trapped, you begin to wonder, "How do I get out of this place?"

On one hand, you are pure potential and you *know* this. On the other hand, your beliefs of not being enough or being unworthy are limiting you. You're serving two masters. It's like a war inside. So how to shift to serving just the true one, right?

You are never upset, afraid, depressed, worried, anxious, sad, or angry for the reason you think. Almost every immediate emotional reaction is a surface reaction rooted deeply in an experience from our past where we separated from our Source, played small, or shifted in some way to survive in the moment, but didn't return. There's still a little piece of us waiting to return and every time we have a trigger, it's an opportunity to see, recognize, and honor ourselves by returning to that highest potential.

Yogah Chitta Vritti Nirodahah— Yoga Sutra 1.2 (Yoga is the union of consciousness within you) reminds us that from our truest expansion, we have experienced a contraction and separation from our Truth.

You didn't get to where you are now without years, maybe decades of conditioning. I can assure you, there are only a limited number of the roots of separation. Once you identify them, it's easy to recognize how far and wide those roots spread. Lovingly, one by one, follow them to the source and gently return to the place where you got off course originally. And yes, your mind playing GPS is going to lead you astray over and over and over in attempt to 'protect' you. Sometimes the GPS software needs updating as paths change. That's what yoga does.

Returning to your Truth becomes easier and easier with much shorter delays and far less painful setbacks. As you begin to say yes to yourself, follow those roots and lovingly return to the space of pure consciousness, you build self-trust. If you trust yourself, you are more likely to take the risk of loving yourself enough to show up fully. You begin to accept all pieces of yourself. That is pure strength when fear and doubt no longer hold you back from showing up fully as the brilliant being you are.

Physical strength is often confused with inner fortitude and fear. Over the years, I've heard "I can't do that" and watched students simply stop, refusing to try because they believed they couldn't do it. This often happens in arm balance and inversion asanas. Maybe you've even thought or said, "I'm not strong enough."

My mom always said, "Can't never could." I'm pretty sure she learned it from her father, a retired U.S. Marine and one of the most resourceful men I ever knew. He didn't make it past the 8th grade, yet he raised two children and one grandchild, maintained a household, and lived seven decades. I don't recall there was anything he couldn't do other than perhaps birth a baby. Can't, in my book, is the "C" word and instantly makes me want to challenge that belief.

There are some things we truly may not be able to do *in the moment*; either we don't know how or we don't have the capacity. Yet, if we are willing to try, we can find a way around or through the limitation to be able to do whatever it is that challenges us. Though I hear, "I can't," the truth is more often, "I won't because I'm scared."

Unwillingness is a safety mechanism. What happens if you try *Bakasana* (crane) and fall forward, hitting your face on the ground? It would likely hurt, but moreover, it would be embarrassing! Humiliation is a show stopper.

When did embarrassment come into the equation of our lives? When we were just toddlers learning to walk, we fell *all the time*! At any point did we stop and think, "Oh, my God! Everyone's watching me! I can't believe I just fell. I'm so humiliated. I'm such an idiot! I'll never do *that* again!" No. Not once.

We saw the big people walking and the goodies were always out of arms reach and crawling was just too slow. So we got back up and tried again and again until walking was possible. Then came running. More falls came of course, but when it worked, there was freedom! Inspired, we kept going. Nothing could stop the progress.

At some point, though, embarrassment and humiliation came into play. Those are game changers. They created the markers in our mind that we judge every potential on and project into the future so we can stay "safe." Is it really safe?

When you step on the mat the first time, you may not have the strength or courage to move out of your safety zone. Through modifications and a willingness to keep showing up, keep leaning into your edges, you start to develop strength - both mental and physical. The more you're willing to try on the mat, the more you become willing to courageously show up and take risks off the mat because you start to trust yourself.

One of my students, Wayne, decided in his late sixties he was going to learn how to do headstands. He practiced and practiced, much to his children's dismay. One day he came into class and kicked up into headstand. The whole class stopped and watched because Wayne was old enough to be a grandfather to just about everyone in class. He did headstands up until about a year before his death- almost a decades worth! What I will always remember about those headstands was his laugh and lingering smile on his face *every single time* he came out of the headstand. He wasn't going to let his fear get him.

As the challenges come off the mat, you begin to realize that you are strong enough to handle it. You become willing to take risks, try new things. You start to find joy in the trying, even if whatever you try doesn't fully pan out as you hoped. Every try is an expansion for your mind and soul. That's freedom.

Life will throw you curveballs. There will be moments when you find yourself wondering if you have the strength to face them, to keep going. In those moments, always return to the breath. Remember a time when you didn't think you could do an asana and discovered you could. Think of how much stronger your asanas became as you kept showing up. All you have to do is show up in each and every moment. When it's too much, return to the breath.

You are stronger than you know. Just believe, breathe, show up, take the risk. If it doesn't work out, you know you tried. Just get back up and try again, only this time, apply what you learned from what was working and build on that. This is true strength.

Toolbox

Asana:

Virabadrasana I

With the feet together, take a large enough step back that your front knee when bent, is over the ankle, and not so large that the back heel can't come close to the ground. The back foot will angle out 45 degrees (or more depending on flexibility). Your front knee bends. Both hips and shoulder are optimally facing forward. Reach your arms up overhead, palms facing one another. Hold for five breaths.

Courage warrior version

Hold each arm position for 3-5 breaths and notice how you feel.

Connected/disarmed Warrior: Arms down by sides of body, palms facing forward.

Giving warrior: Arms extended to the front, slightly below shoulder height, palms up.

Receiving warrior: Arms extended out to the sides, even with shoulders, palms up.

Victorious warrior: Arms overhead and wider than shoulder distance, palms facing each other, chest lifted slightly
Humble warrior: Hands clasped behind the back, bow forward taking shoulder to inside of front knee, lift hands toward ceiling/sky.

Swadhyaya:

Courage to be you

When doing *Virabadrasana* I, you face forward, heart is completely exposed. When you show up unapologetically authentic, you risk vulnerability. It takes courage to show up fully. Courage is also required to disarm ego and pride, speak your truth, admit when you're wrong, ask forgiveness and seek your needs. What fear outweighs your courage? What would you need to be more courageous on a daily basis?

Dropping the judgment

Virabadrasana I teaches us that to show up fully, you absolutely have to be willing to drop your judgment on yourself and the fear of being judged. One of the most powerful lessons I ever learned was when my friend, Sean, said, "What other people think of you is none of your damn business!" In what ways are you judging yourself? What would allow you the freedom to release that judgement? What would happen if you dropped your judgment of others?

Breath:

Inhaling deeply through the nose, exhale slowly and softly through the mouth like you're blowing a butterfly off your body.

Mudra:

Mushti

Bend the four fingers touching the tips lightly to the palm. Rest the thumb over the ring finger. This mudra promotes digestion and reduces aggressiveness and anger.

Mantra:

I am courageous, confident, and clear.

Balance

Balance is equilibrium. On the mat, balance typically refers to simply being able to hold the asana without wobbling or falling over. Off the mat, it's about being able to engage in all areas of your life from a place of equilibrium; one or two areas do not over consume time, energy, or effort at the cost of other highly valued areas. I think most people come to yoga in a place of imbalance- physically, mentally, emotionally, and/or spiritually. I know I did.

I lived the first four decades of my life with a closed-off, protected heart. I was pretty convinced everyone I loved would leave, literally or emotionally. I became obsessed with "heart openers" in my early career. Those openers, I have no doubt, is what finally helped me see that the only person who had been abandoning me was me — in so many ways I would hold back, play small, self-sabotage to avoid losing what I so desired, I simply wouldn't ever fully invest enough to receive it.

I remember one of those heart opening classes that I led quite vividly. The opening meditation was:

Love is expressed through Consciousness. Use your temple, your human body, to expand Consciousness so that you can truly see what Is. The physical eye cannot see this vision, only the soul can see it. Care for your body with love and respect. It is your vehicle in this life to achieve your unique expression of Love. Therefore, Consciousness within us, creator of all that is good, beautiful, and holy, do not forget us. Remind us daily of our Love.

As we moved through the beginning, I asked, "How do you seek the good, beautiful, and holy? How do you create it in your life? How do you share it with others?"

I took the class through a series of heart opening backbends. "Listen to your heart, take inspired action based on your heart. That inspired action is how we use the body to expand into greater love. Jesus commanded his followers, 'Love your neighbors as you love yourself.' Seek to see none as separate from yourself. See clearly the actions rooted in a place of separation, not from their purest essence that is perfect, like you, me and everyone."

As we moved through the sun salutations, I said, "Energy flows where focus goes. Let your heart start guiding you. The more you do, the more it remembers."

As we moved into *Virabadrasana* (Warrior) II, I said, "Here, in this pose, the back of your body is reaching to the back of the mat, your past. You know what you know. You've experienced what you've experienced. While the front half of the body is reaching toward the front of the mat, or the future. Your gaze is set forward, your third eye (center of the forehead just above bridge of nose) paying attention to what lies ahead. But, your mind is behind the third eye. Your throat, where you speak your truth, is over your heart. Your heart is over your solar plexus chakra, your power, passion and drive, which is over your sacral chakra, your creativity and sensuality, as well as your root chakra, your identification with safety and security. All major chakras are in the center, balanced in the present. This asana reminds us to be centered. No matter what life hands us, trying to pull us into the past or future, we are wise to stay present."

In your own practice, try doing the Buddhist loving kindness meditation, Metta. Imagine someone you adore in front of you and send your love and gratitude to that person. In your mind's eye, look them in the eye and say, "May you be happy, healthy, free from fear and have perfect peace." See them saying it back to you. Allow your hearts to connect.

When you change to the other side, think of someone who challenges you. I remember to surrender the separation I might feel from this person and see them as their essence, just like I am, a human experiencing the hurts and fears, joys and sorrow, perfectly imperfect. Send them love. In your mind's eye, look them in the eye and repeat the wish, "May you be happy, healthy, free from fear and have perfect peace." Imagine them saying it back to you (this can be challenging, just trust they mean it because it comes from the soul level). Again, the hearts connect.

This is a powerful exercise to transform energy. I have witnessed it both in my life and through the stories students share. The exercise takes us beyond the assumptions we make and the stories we create to a neutral state. One student told me after we did this her boss had always been very dismissive to her, if he acknowledged her. Though nothing had changed at work, the very day we did this practice, her boss came up to her and told her that he'd been meaning to tell her what a great job she'd been doing and he was grateful for her work. I will never forget the awe-inspired confused look on her face as she concluded her story, "Wendy, that exercise we did is the *only* thing that was different. That wasn't even his kind of language. But something shifted and every day since we did it has been easier and more pleasant. Thank you."

Energetically, she moved more into equilibrium. We don't often know the experiences others have had in their lives or how they have been affected by them, particularly the people who challenge us. It is very hard to see through their actions, particularly if those actions are hurtful, that deep down they aren't so different. Like us they want to be safe, accepted, and loved. Seeing through the actions and offering unconditional love makes a crack for Light to shine through, shifting the balance.

We pull ourselves out of balance all the time in the quest to be safe, accepted, and loved while dancing in the shadows of the beliefs about our own worthiness to be loved and accepted. When you get upset, you allow yourself to be pulled from the present, separating yourself from your true nature, which is pure Light and Love. With curiosity and wonder, ask yourself what you are really upset about, what needs to shift into creating what is good, beautiful, and holy. What needs to shift to expand the perception of love? Are you willing to go there?

Curiosity allows a state of being rather than doing. You're just exploring. There's nothing to change or fix, so it is safe. When I discovered this wondrous exploration, I was in a place where I was really struggling. Living in a very remote rural location, our internet was spotty at best. The inability to connect was costing me time and business. I was angry and frustrated.

What was really upsetting me though was the inability to communicate with clients, potential clients, friends. As I explored this, I realized there was more about communication than just the internet. I recognized that I struggled to talk to my partner about certain topics. Communicating my gifts with others also always came up short. There were layers around communication that I'd never really realized until I started exploring.

As I explored further, I felt the depth of shame and guilt arise about not being where I wanted to be in life. I saw a vast amount of expectations I had put on myself and failed to meet. I saw all the ways I tried to control everything, as well as all the ways I self-sabotaged myself in order to stay safe, accepted, and loved. I'd become my own biggest enemy!

What I was creating was the opposite of good, beautiful, or holy. I asked my guides, angels, the Divine to help me shift my perspective because I believed I didn't know how. However, I sensed that if I'd created these limitations, I could create something different. I didn't know *how*, but I was willing. I was grateful for this awareness and insight.

You don't have to "know how." That's a mind thing and the mind's number one objective is to keep you safe, so it makes you believe you don't know. Just be willing to shift the equilibrium. You will be guided in interesting ways. A book, article, song, or post will happen at just the right moment. A friend will show up unexpectedly and share just what you need to hear. You'll just *feel* like you need to do something. In all cases, they are leading you closer to yourself and your state of balance.

Believing you don't know how implies imperfection. We are perfect. You, me, the trees, the animals, the people around us (even when they aren't acting in a way we'd consider perfect). Perfect. Nothing can change this. You, however, can CHOOSE to not believe this. Fear and doubt exists anywhere that there is an absence of love. Suffice to say, if you are wrestling with fear and doubt, you're not in the spirit of love — for yourself, for others. In and of itself, that's perfect because you're experiencing a place to expand from the illusion. The question is, are you ready to evolve this particular perfection?

Over the years when I have shared this, I am often met with the response, "I need a miracle!" Miracles cannot be performed in the spirit of fear and doubt. Notice how you feel physically when you're in the place of fear and doubt versus when you feel great. How do you treat yourself? Do you eat right and exercise, have a bunch of mind blowing sex? Not likely.

If the body is a temple to hold the essence or energy of love, then the holiness is the altar inside the temple. That's where the true beauty lies. The temple responds to the belief in fear and doubt, the pain of separation. If someone is bringing their shit to dump in the temple, the temple won't be so pretty anymore, will it?

The spirit was before the body. Therefore, the mind is what is creating the reality around you and the body is simply a learning device for the mind. Personally, I know every injury and illness I have suffered has been of my own creation. When my ingestion, digestion, assimilation, or elimination of everything physical, mental, and emotional that I take in is balanced, my immune system and body stay strong and optimal. I can only know what is true for me and this is my truth.

That's all there is, really, when it comes right down to it. We're all here to be the vessel for Love. All the imbalance is nothing more than contrast for what Is, our Truth. We have to allow ourselves to be guided. Trust that you are sharing what you most need. To get love, you give love.

Have you ever lost your balance in an asana? I see this a lot in *Virkasana*, or tree pose. The full expression of the pose is to have one foot high upon the inner thigh of the supporting leg. A modified and far more stable version is to keep the ball of the foot on the floor with the heel resting above the inner ankle of the supporting leg. Students will aim for the full expression repeatedly, even when imbalanced. All they have to do is come to *Tadasana*, mountain pose, take a breath and move into a more modified version where they can practice developing confidence and balance. Yet, they don't.

Life will throw us off balance. We can try to force our way through or we can stop and regroup and explore what is needed in that moment. That brings balance.

Fear arises every time you truly want something that conflicts with your actions. That is imbalance. If you want greatness, but you doubt your worthiness, you're going to be afraid of all the 'what if's'. When you have fear, pay attention and shift it as soon as you become aware of it. No one can do it for you.

Conflict is an expression of fear. Fear arises from a lack of love. The only remedy is unconditional love. All thinking produces form at some level. Thoughts become words, words become actions, actions create beliefs. BAM! Fear or love, you choose.

If you have spent decades in this scarcity, fear-based way of thinking and living, shifting can feel overwhelming. Sort of like committing to clean out a garage after years of shoving shit in it. First, you take everything out onto the driveway. You look at all the stuff and ask, "What in all of this is good? What is holy or pure?" Think about your life, right now. What falls into those categories?

Whatever you come up with, even if it's just a couple of things, is what you keep because they were co-created with the Divine. Everything else, toss it. Put it to the curb. It does not serve you. You no longer need it. Spring clean that crap, baby!

The mind creates fear and scarcity; from that space, 'evil' seems real. Hurt people hurt; they hurt themselves, others, and often both. Take a look around and see what we've created. Wars, disease, famine, abuse. Vicious. Dr Martin Luther King, Jr. once talked about light overcoming darkness and love overcoming hate. I believe that is true.

Test this out for yourself. Look at the little 'evils' in your life — the way your boss treats you at work, money struggles, your relationship with a family member, whatever. Try fighting it, being angry about it, withhold your love from it. Give it a few days. See how *you* feel. See what happens with the situation. Then pivot for a week. Bring some love to it. Even if you think they are wrong for what they've done or doubt anything could change, it's just an experiment. Love them with everything you've got. I find it helps to focus on a person's essence, that pure place inside of them that they protect from hurt, just like you and I do with ourselves. See what changes.

Balance is a return to love and peace. When you surrender everything that has affected your equilibrium, you can be balanced in a state of flow and joy. Because we choose the Divine Play, limitations will tug at our balance from time to time. It's your choice how long you want to stay there. Root into the earth, reach towards the sun and the moon and breathe in the perfection of the present moment. Balance.

Toolbox

Asana:

Virkasana

Stand with feet parallel and a few inches apart. Bring palms to touch in front of heart. Connect to the four corners of the bottom of each foot by lifting and spreading the toes before lightly returning to floor. Shift weight onto one leg. Lift the other foot and place ball of foot on floor, heel resting above ankle on supporting leg, or on the inner calf of supporting leg or inner thigh of supporting leg.

Lift arms overhead and separate hands shoulder distance apart. Hold for 3-5 breaths. Return hands in front of heart center before lowering foot.

Virabadrasana II

Turn to face the side of your mat and step the feet apart, approximately three feet or under the wrists if you extend arms straight out to the side from the shoulders. Turn one foot to face the front of the mat. This is now the "front" foot. The heel should be in a line with the ball or the arch of the back foot. Bend the front knee, aiming to bring the knee over the ankle, but not beyond the ankle. Extend the arms to the sides, straight out from the shoulder. Hips are even (the front hip will often try to drop), ribs over the hips, shoulder over the ribs. Allow the shoulders to soften and look out over your front hand.

Swadhyaya:

Balance. How easy is it for you to fall out of balance? Are you able to set healthy boundaries for yourself? What would your life being in balance look like? Feel like? What needs to shift in order for that to happen?

<u>Metta</u>

This simple Buddhist meditation is so lovely to practice in *Virabadrasana* II. Pick 3 people: someone you adore, an acquaintance you are friendly with, and someone who challenges you. In all three cases, imagine being able to see through them to their soul. Are you able to see the parts of them that have hurt like you have? From a place of compassion (and love), one at a time, wish them:

May you be happy.

May you be healthy.

May you be free from fear.

May you have peace.

Imagine each wishing that back to you. As they do, your hearts connect with a beautiful silvery, white light. Try expanding this outward to your community, the planet, other people.

Breath:

Nadi Shodhana

Use Vishnu mudra to facilitate the passage of air through the nostrils: Bend the first two fingers of the right hand into the palm, using the thumb to control the passage of breath through the right nostril and the ring (or third) finger to control the passage of breath through the left nostril. At the beginning, it is important to equalize your ability to inhale and exhale, using a ratio of 1:1, without retention. Exhale through both nostrils. Block the right nostril and inhale slowly through the left. Block the left nostril and exhale slowly through the right. Slowly inhale through the right, block the right nostril and exhale slowly through the left. That is one round.

Mudra:

Hakini

(shown with Virkasana in photo above) Bring palms to touch in front of heart center. Keep the outer edges from pinky fingers to base of palms and thumbs together while pulling the center of the palm, ring, middle and index fingers apart. It makes a lotus flower. Excellent for balancing the heart, opening to compassion. It reminds me a bit of blossoming trees in spring when used during *Virkasana.*

Mantra:

I am worthy. I matter.

Wendy Reese Hartmann

Ishvara Pranidhana — Surrender

We give meaning to everything. Our mind indexes everything based on meaning in order to make sense of the experience. The mind then defines our illusion; safe, joyous, painful, risky, sad, neutral, harmful. The problem is that the true meaning resides within the Great Mystery. We are all a part of that Great Mystery and within our *soul* we contain the knowing of the meaning. The mind is like an outsider looking in, trying to serve as a good soldier, connecting the dots and creating patterns or *samskaras.*

Look at all the things you give meaning to throughout your day. Right now, look around you. That table, wall, person. You've given each meaning. When you experience something pleasurable, you define it as "good." When something doesn't go your way, you give the meaning of bad. However, both are merely your perception and not the Truth.

It is easy to become frustrated and defeated when you start realizing how much meaning you assign to everything. I remember playing with this concept, trying to increase my awareness of my own meaning-making. On one particularly challenging day, I couldn't help but wonder— why does life feel so hard? If I give everything meaning, why on earth would I choose to be frustrated?

"Surrender," The Voice in my heart said calmly, peacefully.

For once, I didn't ask how. I just surrendered. I closed my laptop, walked over and curled up next to my sweetheart. He put his work away and curled up with me. The rest of the night was just about being present, laughing, and loving. Nothing left to do or change, I just needed to be myself, which is perfect. The ease flowed finally. The next day my work flowed more easily.

That's how surrender works. We all resist it with, "Yeah, but *how*?!" and yet every night we still manage to drop into slumber. You just decide to quit pushing, forcing, or trying to make it happen. You lean in and ask for some Divine guidance or remembrance. You engage faith, trusting yourself and the wisdom enough to allow it to play out as it chooses.

This doesn't mean you sit back and think "all I have to do is surrender" and the world will come to you. We are co-creators. What we surrender are the *kanchukas* (excuses), *kleshas* (shadows), scarcity and separation beliefs. We return with wonder and curiosity to possibilities.

Not knowing "how" ceases to matter as we try to figure out what we do know and where that will take us. We surrender our need for control and are given a buffet of options.

Within each asana, we can fight to be perfect or we can surrender into the experience. The breath provides freedom to lengthen, deepen, and soften. When we surrender the need to be the best (or even as good as) someone else, we can simply be ourselves which is always enough. Good lesson off the mat, too. Look, everyone drinks, sleeps, and farts (sometimes in class, even). Regardless of how close you get to the fullest expression of an asana, everyone gets the same benefits from doing the asana. In that way, we're all equal.

When I practice in a place of surrender and acceptance, I find myself smiling. My practice just *feels* better. On the teacher's mat, I see the struggle. The concentration of the students trying to do the asana just detracts so from the possible joy available within the asana.

I remember one particular class trying to get people to smile. One person was so resistant that it tickled me. Nothing, and I mean nothing, was going to make this person smile. After class, the person approached me and said their job required them to be "happy and on" all the time and this was the one place they didn't have to be. Something about that felt very sad to me. Why did it have to be an either/or?

When you have to force yourself to be joyful in your work and life, it's definitely time to surrender. Your actions then are not congruent with your true nature. Yoga will always show us the imbalance, inflexibility, and weak spots in our life. The question is, will you surrender or will you keep trying to force your way through?

Savasana teaches integration through surrender. It is the last pose in a yoga class. "Corpse pose" allows us to drop into the silence, let the work of the practice settle in, and surrender what no longer serves us so that what is ready to come through may be birthed.

Creating moments of quiet to allow surrender helps us to align with our Highest Self. If we are in the middle of a particularly challenging situation, we can sense how we *want* to feel. We can see where we are forcing or resisting and choose to shift. Doing this offers the possibility for experiencing ease, the path of least resistance. Many people describe this as a state of flow, where energy just moves through us and directs us to where we need to be, when we need to be there, with whom we need to be.

Surrendering is always a choice. Regardless of what is happening, we can choose how we want to show up and play in the energy. We can resist, force, take things personally, or we can surrender and re-align to what our hearts truly desire.

It took many years before I finally surrendered. When I did, yoga took to me to a deeper level of remembrance; why I am here, the Divine Play, and the soul agreements I'd made. There'd always been a longing, like there was something more that I felt yoga wanted to offer, but I couldn't quite attain it.

I needed to surrender. Like a flower blossoming, my world opened up to a whole new dimension I would not have been willing to explore previous to the surrender. I was too busy trying to control my life to recognize nothing was controllable. Surrender gave me freedom, the "something more" my soul had been craving.

Part 2

Divine Play

Once I surrendered, the deeper exploration began. Who am I? That was easy: a divine, infinite being, part of the Great Mystery, but not the Great Mystery itself. Rather, a way for the Great Mystery to experience and evolve into a more perfect perfection.

The harder question is why are we here?

Hell if I know.

I'd be lying if I told you definitively I do.

Here's what I *do* know.

There are some really cool stories about Creation. For me, one in particular felt like an awakening the first time I heard it, like having been under water and finally being able to take a breath of air. I had a visceral reaction of, "Yes! That's it!"

I think it's because of all the shit I've heard over the years (and I heard a lot growing up in the belt buckle of the Bible Belt). It was the only one that made sense as to why bad stuff happens. You may struggle with this version, but what the heck? If you can go get absorbed in a movie, completely suspend your sense of belief, and walk out feeling like, "Yeah, that could happen," then you can believe in this myth.

That said, don't take my word for it. I'm just passing it on as I understand it and shape it for my life. Like me, many of the clients and students I have had the honor of sharing this with have found magic and healing in it, too.

Take it. Leave it. Find your own. Morph this. Just find something to believe in and strive to be whole.

Now, the story (in my simplistic version)…

Shiva, the Divine Masculine, and his better half, Shakti, the Divine Feminine, made a conscious decision to inhabit Earth in human form. These two infinite Deities became finite to explore, what I call…

The Rule of 5's:

5 elements

5 senses

5 limitations (kanchukas)

5 shadows (kleshas)

5 "lower" chakras (root, sacral, solar plexus, heart, and throat)

They created an illusion (maya) of "reality" to explore a contraction into the shadows and an expansion back into their BEingness. When you contract into the shadows, you experience the opposite of being infinite; you feel the shadowy emotions of anger, sadness, grief, jealousy, rage, resentment, loss. Take a moment to think of a time when you experienced one (or more) of those emotions. Can you recall how your body literally physically contracted? Now think of a time when you experienced profound beauty or love; a beautiful sunrise or sunset, a child's hug, nature, a moment after a toe-curling orgasm. Your body naturally expands, opening to receive deep breath.

The contraction is called *Lila* or Divine Play. Perhaps this is the earliest form of masochism, the characteristic when a person finds pleasure in self-denial. Perhaps there is more pleasure than we are conscious of within the contraction and experiencing our shadowy emotions. Yet, we always bemoan those challenging times and feelings as bad and long for them to go away.

Each of us have our own unique iteration of how we play in the illusion and separation, though they are all based on the core five.

The five limitations, kanchukas, that make up an illusion are:

1. **Kalaa** — the belief of limited capacity.

2. **Avidya —** the belief of limited knowledge

3. **Raga** — the belief in not "enough"

4. **Kaala** — the belief that time is real and the desire to pull from the past and project into the future

5. **Niyatithat —** the belief in and fear of death.

These are the core excuses that we use to give us the illusion of being safe from the risk of not being accepted or loved. Have you ever said "I can't" when really you were just too afraid of being judged to try? Or continually educate yourself instead of showing up and applying your knowledge or wisdom? When and where have you grasped the "not (fill in the blank) enough" belief? Time is a huge excuse for many people and yet we all share the same 24 hours in a day. The more hideous version comes from the moment we decide we never want to experience a difficult or painful experience and our minds create a map that compares every *potential* experience against the painful one and keeps us stuck in order to feel safe against the old pain reoccurring.

The kleshas, or five of the ways the separation or illusion, are:

1. **Purusha**— the Divine spark within all is forgotten
2. **Prakriti**— there are shadow aspects to knowledge: reality, action or passion, and a resistance, ignorance, or procrastination to remembering.
3. **Ahamkara**— comparison leading to judgment
4. **Buddhi**— I-identification
5. **Manas**— distinct perceptions of the mind

These are deeper more subconscious limitations that keep us separated from our Highest Self, our deepest wisdom, to our fullest potential. If these were veils, they would be covering our "inner jewel" as the Buddhists call it.

I am willing to bet you can look back and see how these excuses and shadows have played out in your own life. Likewise, I am willing to bet your life hasn't been total crap either. There've probably been lots and lots of super cool moments as well as really nice, pleasurable, happy moments.

Shiva and Shakti left behind their Divine status when they incarnated in human form to be able to experience the totality of shadow and light. That's where the senses and elements come in.

There are five ways to perceive our experiences.

The five senses:

1. Hearing
2. Touch
3. Sight
4. Taste
5. Smell

The five instruments of action:

1. speaking
2. grasping
3. walking
4. excreting
5. generation

The five elements play into this, too, though we tend to overlook these in our daily living.

1. fire
2. earth
3. air
4. water
5. ether

Shiva embodied action, while Shakti embodied wisdom. Though they were complimentary aspects of one deity, we could consider them the first "Power Couple." Their embodiment into human form to experience the totality of shadow and light is reflected in our own human journey. This takes us to our Soul Plan.

As I mentioned before, embodying as human, contracting into the limitations and shadows, is the Divine Play.

I grew up across the street from a playground. It had two concrete picnic tables with benches, a large slide, monkey bars, "jungle gym," three levels of pull-up bars, a sandbox with a teeter-totter and rocking horses, a swing set, and a merry-go-round. These were the staple "toys" I, or anyone at the playground, could choose. However, how I chose to see them or play on them was uniquely mine.

For example, those picnic tables at the park were at one time or another a classroom, the White House, a spaceship, my stage, my house. I am sure there were more, but these tended to be my favorite iterations. I made them uniquely mine in the moment. That is how life is; we choose our Divine Play.

I can hear the objections now. "Yeah, but that hurt wasn't my fault." You're right. It was part of a contract to experience contrast and allow you the opportunity to evolve. We'll talk about those agreements in the next chapter. Let's look at you first.

For the most part, there is a moment when we realize we cannot shine at our brightest. Perhaps a parent is having a tough day in their own *maya* (illusion) and snaps when their attention is sought. In a moment of confusion from hearing, "Not now, I am busy!" the young brain processes that if attention, adoration, and love is to be received again, then caution needs to be heeded on the right time and place for showing up. Or a teacher does a lousy job of communicating a correction and the child personalizes it. There are an infinite number of reasons we disconnect. If you take a few moments to close your eyes and breathe steadily, you might remember some times when you sensed it wasn't okay to be the whole version of yourself.

Every moment in our existence creates a *samskara*, or mental impression, that affects us. When we repeat an action or situation, literally or mentally, we create deep grooves in our mind. These grooves, like ruts in mud, can derail us and keep us stuck. In the stuckness, we experience *tamas*, the dark, destructive, chaotic place. It's hard to see a way out of the ruts. It feels heavy and permanent. Limitations and shadows love *tamas*. That's their playground.

Other *samskaras,* like the Divine Masculine, are action oriented. It's a doing. This is rajas, or action. This can be good such as when we are able to push out of the ruts and get started again or take action on righting a wrong. It's where passion meets action. Alternatively, it can be all-consuming and create its own rut of "should's" and "have-to's" in order to feel safe, accepted, and loved. It's at the heart of burn out. *Rajas* is the fire. Fire can warm and create transformation (think cooking) or fire can burn and consume (think forest fire).

If, however, you can see the limitations and shadows for what they are, your *samskara* becomes *sattvic*, or conscious. *Sattva* is constructive, harmonious, and goodness. Too much *sattva* and it's hard to exist in the world. You'd rather run off to a cave and meditate to be with God. You are, after all, here for Divine Play which means getting a little messy.

There is a wonderful movie that illustrates this Divine Play called *Michael*, starring John Travolta as Archangel Michael. The story is about Michael's last journey to Earth. He's got one more mission. However, while on that mission, he's committed whole-heartedly to playing in the limitations— he smokes, drinks, eats pounds of sugar, challenges bulls, flirts with women, and dances. He knows he's going home and there's nothing he can do about that, so while on this final mission (I won't give everything away if you haven't seen it,) he's going to live it up and "smell the roses."

That's Divine Play. We contract. We expand. We engage the five sense and five elements. There are moments of profound pain and sheer bliss. We have orgasms for goodness sake (pun intended). We are naughty and nice. We feel each other's fear, pain, doubt, because we can. We don't have to. Ask a sociopath about empathy; they have none. The Divine Play, as twisted as this may sound, is *fun* for our soul and necessary for our evolution!

Yep, I hear ya. But how is watching a loved one die fun? How is heartbreak fun? How is injustice fun? In the literal sense, it's not. It takes us to the depths of our shadows. There will come a time when we look back with the hindsight of a God and think, "That wasn't so bad." In the moment though it sucks.

There's another layer in the Divine Play— archetypes.

At those picnic tables, I was a mom, teacher, chef, US President, performing artist, star of the show. They were roles I played. The archetypes are role models we play with to experience the shadows and light. The archetypes are actually energetically neutral. We give them their meaning and energetic charge, positive or negative.

All of us share four core archetypes—child, victim, saboteur, and prostitute. At first glance, they may look really negative just by their names. You can't judge an archetype by its name.

The core archetypes determine how we:

- choose to survive
- remain separated from Source
- return to Source
- relate to material world

- respond to authority
- make choices and show up in relationships, even the most important relationship—the one with your Self.

The shadow aspect is the separation from consciousness. The shadow aspects are all the ways you played small in order to survive, be loved, feel accepted or safe. Ironically, your shadows are fed by a paradoxical relationship to power—you use them to get something you need, even when that doesn't seem apparent. In other words, there's a payoff for everything you do, even when it seems like you're not getting anything out of them. You are.

For example, when the child is playing in the shadow it needs a sense of safety, security, belonging, and love. If your child is pushing someone away when you really want to be loved, it's like a kid testing parental boundaries in real life, right? The victim will play in the shadows to not have to take responsibility. The saboteur will keep you playing small to avoid the pain of being hurt. The prostitute will play in the shadows to make up for your lack of faith and trust in your highest Self. The shadow play contains the secret reason for self-sabotaging opportunities.

The shadow aspects come into play when you avoid feelings, repressing them for fear of consequences. An example is when someone oversteps a boundary and you feel anger, but you repress the anger for fear of being abandoned, judged, criticized, hurt, or punished. We are forced into the shadows when we choose to be ignorant of acting from fear.

When you decide to confront these shadow aspects, you are committing to change. The mind recognizes change as a loss of control. That loops back to the map of fear of isolation, that you'll lose the people you love because you're being vulnerable, even though they love you because of your vulnerability. Additionally, there is a fear of taking responsibility. That fear paralyzes many people.

Facing your shadow is often not fun. In fact, it can be scary! Just remember, we are facing our shadows together. While the work is yours alone, you are not alone. You have a safe space to return to in order to share, vent, ask, cry, celebrate, and simply show up as you. I believe with all my heart and soul that you are a Divine, infinite being and you are ready to remember that Divinity.

I want to give a brief overview of each of the archetypes.

The **child** helps us connect to safety, security, and belonging. In the light, this archetype is connected to innocence, nature, creativity, and curiosity. In the shadow, it is needy, temperamental, depressed, fearful, might hide, and can even be obnoxious with distractions and meltdowns.

The **saboteur** reminds us of our strength, courage, and trusting our intuition. In the light it helps us to break through false beliefs and take action. In the shadow, it creates disruption, resists opportunities, brings up all the false beliefs based on the foundation of our illusion created when we started playing small.

The **victim** helps us with boundaries, particularly around power. In the light, it helps us with self-esteem and personal power. In the shadows, it manipulates, creates excuses, earns sympathy.

The **prostitute** is our connection to faith that we are supported, nurtured, and loved because we are Divine. In the light, it helps us with the moral compass of what we are willing to exchange for safety, security, belonging, and love. In the shadows, it will do what it has to do to survive.

There are eight other archetypes that are unique to each person's soul plan. The twelve total archetypes each live in their own "house." If you could make a feng shui grid on that playground, these would be the houses: personality/ego, life values, self-expression, creativity and prosperity, career and health, relationships, outside resources, spirituality, your place in the world, highest potential, and unconscious. These twelve houses correspond to the astrological signs that are themselves archetypal expressions.

As you can see, this is no ordinary playground. We play here to experience the richness, the moist and dark places, the dry and desolate places, and everything at our essence that we are not. Just like people with curly hair want straight hair or vice versa, short people want to be tall, skinny people want to be muscular. We want what we don't have because we want to play in the totality of possibilities.

The best part of the lila (play) is the maya (the illusion). Honestly, I don't know how much we can transcend the maya while in human form, but then again, isn't that a limitation in and of itself? I wonder sometimes if we'd really want to transcend all limitations. As a species, we haven't exactly evolved out of the crabs in a bucket mentality. If someone did figure out how to break through all limitations of their mind, create spontaneous healing, raise the dead, turn water into wine… oh, wait. Someone did do that. Yeah, that didn't turn out so well for that person.

All joking aside, what if it's just about finding the silliness in it all? Dancing in and out of the shadows and light, experiencing the richness and having fun even with the contractions within our maya? Wouldn't that be extremely liberating?

Sacred Agreements + Soul Plans

As you start to dig into the deeper questions of "who am I and why am I here?", it's important to know about soul plans and agreements.

From *my* human form, I like to imagine it went a little like happy hour at my favorite wine bar…

There is a group of friends sitting around the table discussing Divine qualities such as love, compassion, truth, justice, creation, and acceptance. Each embodies more of certain qualities than others. The common thread is a desired experience in the *totality* of the quality, both the shadow and light aspects. These are, after all, Divine and infinite Beings, sans limitations. What more fun than to play in the opposite of your average, everyday experience?

In order for these divine infinite beings to truly experience the totality they'd have to become limited.

Now, as it always happens, some of the friends had more experience than others. They knew what it meant to become limited. Even if they tried to convince the less experienced, it wouldn't matter. There's a belief, even there that what happens to someone else, won't happen to you. And even in the Beyond, excitement and creativity is contagious.

So when one gets really excited about a quality they are ready to go for and starts asking for help, the more experienced groan a bit but are willing to abide and choose their roles carefully. The less experienced shimmer with anticipation and decide to, as we say, "go big or go home".

They were, quite frankly, tired of "home" and wanted a change of pace. It does get a little boring when you have absolutely everything you want. Far more fun when you *can't* get what you want, when you have to really work at it. Oh, and even more exciting when you forget you have the power to change it.

The less experienced started drilling the more experienced with questions. Illusion, what humans call reality, is always far stranger than even an infinite being can comprehend. While every illusion is a little different, there are some common rules everyone has to follow:

1. Before your tenth year in human form, your illusion will be in full effect,

2. The Rule of Fives,

3. The only two things you absolutely have to do are die and change (both are inevitable),

4. Where and how you play, though you may not believe it while in the illusion, is your choice,

5. All you have to do to dissolve the illusion is ask for help and be willing.

The less experienced would go fully into their illusion sooner than a more experienced being would. The illusion is set the moment a disconnection from essence is experienced. In other words, that moment when being their brightest, most amazing version stopped out of fear of not being loved, accepted, or safe. The illusion takes us into a contracted version of our full self, our Highest Self. If we shut down those parts long enough, we forget the totality. That's where the Divine play really begins to get juicy.

All of us are made up of feminine and masculine energies with the primal powers of will, knowledge, and action. By having chosen a gender for the human body, you can see how one of the powers could be minimized. The power of will is so much more than will-power; it envelopes desire, determination, and impetus. The power of knowledge is the innate within. The power of action is the ability to bring all powers present and to engage what humans call miracles.

Based on your particular plan and the core limitations you choose to experience, disconnection from your essence could occur from a subtle experience or a more traumatic experience. The illusion brings opportunities through the *kanchukas* (excuses) and *kleshas* (shadows) to validate the disconnection, which engrains into thoughts, beliefs, and even actions.

This is Divine play. This is how we spirits get to come play in the limitations and thereby experience the totality of the Divine qualities. This is life. Dancing in and out of the shadows and light. We can't play alone. Remember, we made some agreements to help us on our plan.

Make no mistake, every single being you encounter—from the briefest moment to the most intimate relationship— has an agreement with you.

The four most common agreements are:

Neutral

Limitations Only

Expansion Only

Contraction—Expansion.

Let's start with neutral agreements. These people can swing either way in how you interact. It could be someone who does something nice intentionally and makes you expand or the opposite. Their actions may have no intention behind them at all, but your reaction to them pulls you into contraction or expansion. These are little neutral reminders of how we are here to play.

It could be a barista or waitstaff at a local cafe, the person driving in front of you, the man who opens the door for you, or the person who isn't paying attention and bumps into you causing you to lose your balance and drop what you were carrying. There really is no rhyme or reason with these people. Sometimes you pass someone and have the strangest sensation that you know them, though you know you've never met. That's a neutral contract.

The Limitations Only agreements are hard. Real hard. They could be as long term as an abusive relationship or a situation that in the moment creates a limitation that deepens our dance in the shadows. It could be that uninsured motorist who causes a car accident that physically harms you. It could be the mugger that steals your purse out of your car while you're literally five feet away (true story). It could be the adult who physically, emotionally, or sexually abuses you. In all cases, this person is there to pull you into the limitations, but will not be helping you out of them.

The tricky thing with these is understanding that the agreement to contract you was made out of a place of love, in agreement with an experience you desired in this lifetime. As a human, even knowing what I know, this still sucks and is hard to comprehend. There's a lot of ugly and dark energy around it and it's hard to see in the shadows that there was ever a moment of light around this agreement.

The Expansion Only agreements are the people who see your essence, your potential, and help you remember your greatness. They cheerlead, hold you accountable, call you on your excuses, hold you to a higher standard, inspire and motivate you. They don't play in the limitations with you because they don't need to. They may be teachers, mentors, co-workers, special friends. They may even be coaches, counselors, doctors, or someone you follow but don't know.

The Contractions-Expansions can be seen in most of our relationships, especially friends, family, and lovers. These are the relationships that make us want to be better people while also bringing out the less optimal version of ourselves. They are challenging and inspirational, trying and touching, loving and frustrating. They reflect the best and worst in us. They take us into the limitations and help to remind us of who we really are at the core.

Remember, we come here to play in the limitations, not stay in the limitations. Because we forget when we separate, sometimes it's hard to look objectively at a situation when someone is triggering you into the shadows. We start by noticing how we feel in the moment we are triggered.

I remember one particular visit with my mom; I was pushing her to be outside, go for walks in the forest near my home. She went into the limitation of pain. This triggered in me all the memories of all the things she couldn't do throughout my life because it "hurt too much" or was "too hard." My perception was that she'd hidden behind that excuse her whole life in order to get the attention and love she desired. In that moment, it had the absolute opposite effect on me. It brought up all of the rage, frustration, disappointment I'd carried for so long.

I could not separate the past from the present and allow her to feel what she felt in that moment. I didn't trust her. I didn't accept her as anything other than a victim of her own choosing. Because she'd played that role for so long, I was having to face my own limitations of being intolerant and impatient, a person who was not compassionate or loving unconditionally. We fed each other's limitations.

She told me later, "I know you love me and want the best for me, but this is *my* life. You need to let me live it." I decided then to do just that. Whatever she chose, whether I agreed or not, it was her choice and I would accept it as such.

If she continued to make lifestyle choices that further deteriorated her health that would be her choice. She could not expect me to sympathize about the outcomes. A year later, she called, panicked, when she'd received results of some medical tests.

"Wow. That really sucks. I am truly sorry to hear that," I said.

"Me, too."

"Well, what are you going to do?" I asked

"I have to change."

"Okay, how will you do that?"

"I have to start exercising and eating better."

"True. What specifically will you do?"

"I don't know."

"I am sure you'll figure it out." I wasn't sure at all. The worst part of this conversation was that I was health coaching clients who had received the *exact diagnosis* she had. I knew the answers and she knew I knew. But I kept my commitment. This was her life and I had to let her live it. It wasn't what she was wanting or needing from me.

She wanted to know she was loved, someone was willing to take care of her, which meant they cared. The problem with that was I'd been trying to do just that most of my life. I didn't have to anymore. I could love her without having to save her.

When you are willing to step out of the limitations, yours or others, you begin to live authentically. There is a freedom in the grace of authenticity. You can love unconditionally and refuse to play in the limitations. In fact, loving unconditionally is precisely why you choose not to validate or even destroy the limitations. This is a bold and courageous choice because there is no room for growth, expansion, or authenticity in an imbalanced relationship where one party chooses to remain a victim. If they are unable to be justified and satisfy their needs of support, love, and understanding, they will seek their needs elsewhere. Loss is a challenge for everyone, even when the loss is perhaps the most beneficial outcome.

Interestingly, what I have come to intimately know is that when you make the choice to create authentically and destroy the illusion, even though some relationships end, the quality of each new relationship is much more rewarding.

She made a choice to take control of her health in that moment. Tearfully she said, "I have wanted to die my whole life and I realize now that I'm not ready to die."

We do funny things when we separate from ourselves. All the unworthiness, self-loathing, and playing fully in the illusion of limitations make us hate our life, makes us want to go home because this pain sucks.

We forget those hardships, challenges, and limitations are exactly why we're here, along with the opportunity to move through them and experience the richness and delights of being human. Loving unconditionally is still the most authentic expression you have in this life. It's why we are here. To love the loveless, the oppressed, the hurt.

Because of that love, there is room to say, "I don't want to play this way anymore with this person who triggers me" *and* still love that person. This is creating the space of grace for them to make their own choice to break free or move on to someone else who will play small with them—misery does love company. Ultimately, the person you love deepest, most unconditionally when you make the choice to be authentic, is yourself. You deserve that love. We all do. Expanding into the love out of the limitations is why we play here.

Wendy Reese Hartmann

BEing

I think just about everyone I've encountered, including myself, that adopts the philosophy about Divine Play, Soul Plans and agreements share a common fear. If we actually moved through our contraction, will we have learned all there is to learn? And if so, does that mean we'll die, because what's the point of being here if we're not growing?

Well, I don't really know the answer, but I know that the question is a limitation in and of itself. I do believe there is a way to play in the contrast without getting stuck there, expand and then create new contrasts, repeating as long as we desire. Each expansion takes us beyond our expectations and each, therefore, is growth. In this way, we cease to be limited by the limitations that we choose. Rather, we use each as a contrast and experience the totality, shadow and light.

When we get to this level of Play, our relationships transform profoundly. We don't play in the shadows of blame, shame, and guilt. We don't expect others to make us happy or fulfill us. We can love unconditionally and set healthy boundaries because we know without any doubt that hurt people hurt and those actions do not represent the Divine infinite being, but the soul playing in the contrast.

The contrast reminds us that pain is matter and density manifesting in our bodies in order to validate our subconscious limiting thoughts and beliefs. Thoughts become things and what you resist will persist. For every action there is an equal and opposite reaction because there always has to be balance.

Humans in their limitations are not aligned with the Divine and as long as they are misaligned, they will be a source of friction and act unjustly. It's hard to be here sometimes when you're drowning in the illusion. There's so much pain and suffering all around, much of which seems senseless. And, yes, I get it, we've chosen it. But I watch children dying, terrorists blowing up innocent people, mothers mourning—God that is the worst. I've felt the grief of loss myself. The helpless feeling of not being able to help someone remember their Truth. Ancient temples with beautiful facets of the Truth destroyed—in God's name, no less. The planet has been raped and pillaged in the name of profit. And worse, I've contributed through my own lifestyle. You have too. Natural disasters, sickness, genocide, man-made disasters. There's a lot of pain.

Even reading that, I bet you can feel yourself contracting. We humans are very creative in our limitations.

Yet, I believe in magic and miracles. Love will light the darkness and we are all Love. Returning to Love is a choice that begins with the willingness.

Here, in spite of the illusions we create, there is such beauty. Watching dogs play, hearing children laughing, experiencing toe-curling orgasms, smelling a rose blooming in your garden. I want to surrender my own resistance and feel my lover's arms around me a billion more times, hear my mother and father tell me I am what they are most proud of, watch every sunrise and sunset in full presence. I want to learn how to tango really well, drink wine with friends on the patio under the huge trees in the desert. I want to surf the ocean's waves and in complete presence that offers full freedom. I want to feel the sun on my face, be bathed in warm rain, chase rainbows. I want to read more books and learn more, even if I already know everything (remember, we *are Divine infinite beings)*. There's still so much and I know how much I will miss these experiences when I return to just energy.

What matters most is if we appreciate and utilize our co-creative abilities. Most often we do not because of the illusion. Time to change that. Adopt an attitude of gratitude. Gratitude opens the floodgates to more richness, juiciness, and joy. And that's not just me being a hippy-dippy yoga chick. I'm serious. If you go around focusing on all the shit you don't have you're gonna feel anxious and awful. If you bring overwhelming gratitude for what you do have you find more to be grateful for and that continues to multiply!

I can remember a point in my life when I was struggling hard. Nothing seemed to be working—my health wasn't in a great place and it was affecting my ability to work, so finances stunk, and my relationship was a sham. I remember trying so hard to find something, *anything* to be grateful for in my life. I looked down and saw my sparkly red toenails and thought (and I'm not lying), "I'm grateful to have toenails with a pretty color on them." That's all I had. But you know what? It made me laugh! I realized surely I had something else to be grateful for and within minutes I found a handful of things. I practiced daily, returning to my toenails when I got stuck. Eventually, things shifted. Faster than I expected, actually. I've kept my attitude of gratitude since.

You are now at a pivotal moment in your soul plan. Every moment we have a choice of how we want to see the world. Every moment we have the choice to return to the breath and allow it to guide us back into the present. We realign, find balance, strength, and flexibility. We surrender. We live, fully. That's yoga—union. In the next moment it all begins again. How will you choose?

Live your yoga. Don't just do your yoga. Get calm. Go below the surface. Explore. Digest what you ingest and either assimilate or eliminate. Stay steady. Be fully present with whatever you're creating. Be mindful. Most of the stuff will be concealed, but once it's revealed, whoa! That's the juiciness. Then it begins again. Have fun with it all.

You matter. You are worth this journey. Let us close this with the sound of creation, chanted three times:

Om.

Om.

Om.

It's been an honor and a pleasure to guide you.

Thank you for the opportunity.

Namaste.

In Gratitude

Let's start with every single one of my students—rather you've taken hundreds or simply one of my classes, your energy has taught me. There have been some of you who have asked multiple times, "When are you going to write a book on yoga?" Well, you got it.

I've had many, many yoga teachers over the years only a few standout: Mary Beth Markus and Meg Berlyein of Desert Song Healing Arts Center in Phoenix, Liz Heffernan of Soma Yoga, Rod Stryker and Seane Corn whom I've only had the joy of practicing with a few times in person. Words lack in expressing my infinite love and gratitude for the wisdom and gifts you share.

Ron and Linda Reese, thank you for being life teachers, supporting me, keeping me safe and alive, and providing lovely contrast through the years. Dave Hartmann, I know you have never fully "got" what it is I do, but you've supported me through it all, encouraged me, and loved me in spite of my weird ways. Thank you for creating a safe space for me to be. Thank you for loving me. Thank you for joining me on this journey (finally).

Lorena Streeter, Brianna Renner, Ruth Hirsch, Steve Mattus, Mia Davis, Stacy Ann Clark, Ann Margaret McKillop, Kelly McDermott, Kristi Faust, Jason Stein, Adam Bird, Belen Arriola, Lindsey Radiochini for their help with this process (the latter three for many layers of your help over the years). Nancy Temple aka Photo Mistress, Yoga Goddess, you are the busiest woman I know! Allie Theiss for the final push to make this happen and years of (almost) weekly, "go kick some ass" checks-ins.

And finally, YOU. I may not even know who you are (yet), but I know there's a reason you made it this far. You are magnificent. You matter. You are worthy. You are loved. Integrate your yoga. Listen to your innate wisdom. Be your greatness. It's time. No more kanchukas, okay? The world is waiting for us to show up fully. Let's do this!

Infinite love + gratitude.

About the Author

Yoga chose Wendy Reese Hartmann, not the other way around. After fifteen years, even though she is grateful for the journey, she has yet to figure out why her. She is a 500 hour certified Yoga Teacher that has been teaching since 2001.

Most people describe Wendy Reese Hartmann as weird or wonderful or wonderfully weird depending on if you stick around long enough to get to know her. She adores elephants, rubber ducks, bubbles, sunshine, gardens, magic, good food, dogs playing and being in her kayak on the water. She's still working on being patient, but yoga has gifted her the ability to be calmly tenacious. It is a life mission of hers to surrender the need to take herself so seriously. Some days she's successful.

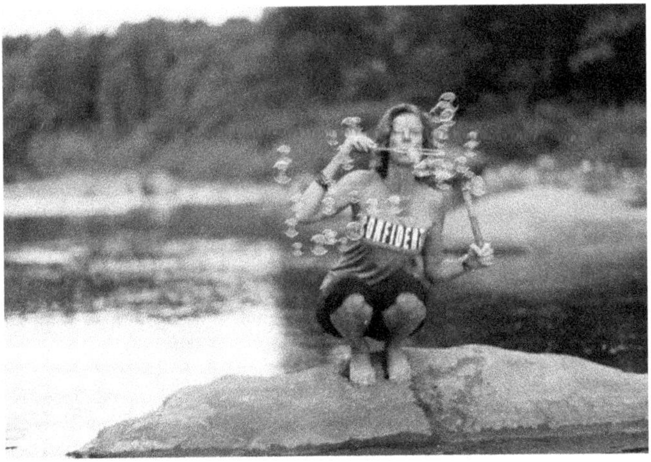

She loves to engage people who are inspired or motivated by her posts, blogs, articles, classes, and books (hint, hint). You can learn more (aka the boring stuff like credentials), engage with Wendy, and receive gifts at www.wholebeinginc.com.

Instagram: @wholebeinginc